The Little
Book of
Mindfulness

'There is nothing either good or bad,
but thinking makes it so.'

Hamlet, Act II

The Little
Book of
Mindfulness

10 Minutes a Day to
Less Stress, More Peace

Dr Patrizia Collard

An Hachette UK Company
www.hachette.co.uk

First published in Great Britain in 2014 by Gaia Books,
a division of Octopus Publishing Group Ltd, Carmelite House,
50 Victoria Embankment, London EC4Y 0DZ
www.octopusbooks.co.uk
www.octopusbooksusa.com

The material in this book was previously published in *Journey into Mindfulness*

Distributed in the US by Hachette Book Group USA,
1290 Avenue of the Americas, 4th and 5th Floors, New York, NY 10104

Distributed in Canada by Canadian Manda Group,
664 Annette St., Toronto, Ontario, Canada M6S 2C8

ISBN 978-1-85675-353-1

A CIP catalogue record for this book
is available from the British Library.

Printed and bound in China
17

Consultant Publisher Liz Dean
Senior Art Editor Juliette Norsworthy
Designer Isabel de Cordova
Illustrations Abigail Read
Production Controller Sarah Kramer

Any information given in
this book is not intended to
be taken as a replacement for
medical advice. Any person
with a condition requiring
medical attention should
consult a qualified practitioner
or therapist. Only practise if
you feel able to. There should
never be pain.

Contents

Introduction

What Is Mindfulness?

Mindfulness is being aware of or bringing attention to this moment in time, deliberately and without judging the experience. So, when we go for a mindful walk (see page 42) we really notice every little detail and all we encounter – trees, cars, flowers growing out of small cracks, or a cat crossing the road – rather than creating to-do lists.

By reconnecting with these simple moments in life, by truly living moment by moment, it is possible to rediscover a sense of peace and enjoyment. We may, at least sometimes, feel once again truly enchanted with life.

As a form of therapy, mindfulness has recently been in the news a great deal. It is recommended by the Department of Health and also in the guidelines set down by NICE (National Institute for Clinical Excellence), and many see it as a cheap, effective and 'doable' intervention for our stress-filled lives, as much as a skill that can prevent us from actually breaking down or becoming ill if we incorporate it into our daily lives.

More than 10,000 published research papers are available on mindfulness-based therapies, should you want to check out the subject in depth, and there are many online videos you can also watch. The application of mindfulness covers a range of situations, such in parenting training, the treatment of mental health, in schools and as part of well-being therapies. It is even used in treating the immune system, with some positive outcomes for patients with HIV, ME (chronic fatigue syndrome) and MS.

Benefits of Practising Mindfulness

People who regularly implement mindfulness strategies may find lasting physical and psychological benefits, such as:
~ Increased experience of calm and relaxation
~ Higher levels of energy and enthusiasm for living
~ Increased self-confidence and self-acceptance
~ Less danger of experiencing stress, depression, anxiety, chronic pain, addiction or low immune efficiency
~ More self-compassion and compassion for others and our planet.

How It Began

Just over 30 years ago, a molecular biologist, while meditating, had the inspiration to bring meditation into the secular world of a hospital. In 1979, Jon Kabat-Zinn gave up his career as a scientist and started a stress-reduction clinic in Massachusetts University Hospital. He had studied Korean Zen and yoga in the past and is a regular meditator.

In the early 1990s, a 40-minute TV programme introduced mindfulness, which originated in contemplative teachings, to a wider audience. Several thousand people wanted to learn the 'mindfulness stuff' after they watched the programme. Around this time Jon wrote

Full Catastrophe Living – the title is based on Alexis Zorbas in the film *Zorba the Greek*, played by Anthony Quinn, who says: 'Am I not a man? And is a man not stupid? I'm a man, so I married. Wife, children, house, everything. The full catastrophe!'

A decade later, psychotherapists in Canada and the UK began to understand that mindfulness interventions may also be useful for reducing and improving psychological disorders. *Mindfulness-Based Cognitive Therapy (MBCT) for Depression* (2002) was the first publication in which the ancient wisdom was interwoven with cognitive therapy to help patients not to relapse into depressive episodes.

Today, MBCT and MBSR (mindfulness-based stress reduction) are used to treat a multitude of illnesses including anxiety, stress, burnout, trauma, chronic pain, some forms of cancer, psoriasis, eating disorders, addiction and obsessive compulsive disorder (OCD).

Learning During a Lunch Hour

In 2008, I wrote an academic paper (Collard and Walsh) that was based on my experience of teaching mindfulness to university employees. The participants were academics, technicians and administration staff. The 'awareness training' that I taught for one lunchtime hour each week was a new set of skills to help the staff achieve a better life–work equilibrium. They were instructed to connect regularly with all their five senses and to focus non-judgementally on the here-and-now experience of life. The exercises I chose were neither difficult to teach nor hard to learn; I did emphasize, however, that students should ideally enter into a regular routine of practice in order for change to occur.

These brief weekly sessions helped to bring about valuable changes and health improvements in the participants. The motto was: we are all different and special, so we do not attempt to become like somebody else, but connect more deeply with our true selves.

Their stress levels were reduced (although Christmas was just round the corner), their language and support for each other became more compassionate and, in general, they felt more joyful and had a sense of life being an adventure.

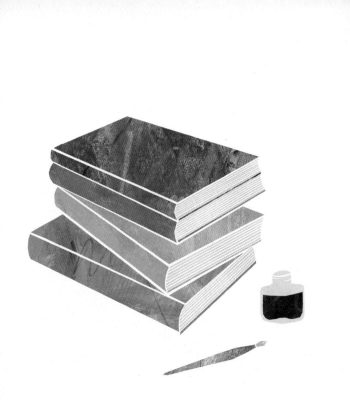

Mindfulness is a new way of being, a
new way of experiencing life and improving
one's work-life balance

Reconnecting to Life

When teaching mindfulness,
we point out that this skill may
not actually 'heal' all ills, but what it will do
is change our perspective on discomfort and
open new possibilities for moving from just 'being'
and 'struggling' back towards 'adventurous living.'
You learn to live around the pain rather than focus
on it all the time. Pain in your shoulder will become
a pain in the shoulder and maybe even retreat into
the background of your awareness while you focus
on the 'breath' or 'listen to sounds around you.'

We have started to understand that mindfulness practice
may prevent us from getting sick and unhappy, but it
can also return our awareness to the childlike curiosity
we all had when we were young. We may experience
once again the wondrous qualities of natural life: a
blade of grass, clouds in the sky, the taste of a delicious
strawberry, the importance of surrounding ourselves
with friends and others who care deeply for us.

We remember all of a sudden that it is these little
moments that are the true wonders of being alive.
These glimpses of joy really matter, because they
connect us to life rather than split us from it.

> 'When you drink just drink,
> when you walk just walk.'

Zen saying

Thoughts Change Our Reality

Mindfulness practice, if regularly observed, can not only
change the biochemistry of our body, but also change the
brain structurally. The title of 'happiest man on earth' has
been given to Matthieu Ricard, a Buddhist monk with a PhD
in biology. He has a much smaller control centre (amygdala)
than other humans and can endure being in an fMRI scanner
for a couple of hours. Once, when he came out of a scanner,
having gone through three long meditations while being
observed, he is supposed to have said that the experience
was almost like a nice retreat. His shrunken amygdala also
helps him not to blink when there is a loud noise close by.
He is 'Mr Calm', but he does still mindfully check a road
before crossing it.

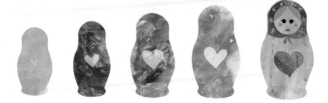

Increasing Gratitude

With this growing of awareness, we subconsciously also increase gratitude and compassion, as can be proven by looking at Functional Magnetic Resonance Imaging (FMRI) studies of the brain.

Appreciation occurs when we begin to realize what we have been gifted with, and loving kindness reconnects us to others in a win–win attitude. We start to focus on positive thoughts and perceptions and, for a while, we let go of our fearful, anxious brain pattern. In fact, every action we engage in can become a daily meditation, a slowing-down and an appreciation of life. It seems so simple, in some ways, that it is almost embarrassing to have to study it.

We need only remember when we were children who gazed at the sky and the drifting clouds. There was nothing to do, nothing to achieve. There was no notion of time nor any guilt for 'wasting' it. Time and guilt are concepts we learn about much later in life.

Join Me...

With this little book, I would like to invite you to join me and feel once more what it is like to be consciously alive and to connect to the sense that every moment of life is precious. I would like to remind you how meaningful it can be to taste a strawberry, or to smell lavender, or to stroke somebody we love and really feel and connect with them.

Of course, as life is a dualistic experience, we will also become more sensitive to the painful aspects of our lives. Yet even this can have advantages. It may prevent us from eating an out-of-date sandwich or staying with a partner or job that is destructive to us. If we all managed to stop doing so much, even for just a few minutes a day, we would enrich our experience of life and help our bodies and minds stay healthy and well.

Each chapter in the book shows you 5- and 10-minute practices and inspirations which you can try in any order that you choose to. You may of course like to take more time to explore them than the times suggested; whatever you do is fine.

My hope and endeavour is to help you move closer to the stillness and joy within.

Meditation and Posture Tips

✳️ Some exercises suggest you sit in a chair. I recommend an upright chair that will support your spine, but is comfortable. It helps to wear loose-fitting clothes and perhaps use a shawl or blanket to prevent you feeling cold – often, when we meditate, we become more relaxed and our body temperature tends to drop a little, just as it does when we get ready for sleep.

✳️ Sit with dignity – neither upright and rigid like a soldier, nor slumping over. Sitting in this way helps you to be focused and aware of any sensation as it arises, and connect with this sensation – temperature, sound, or your breathing, for example – as an anchor of awareness, to prevent your mind roaming and ending up in some anxious train of thought.

✳️ Each time you get ready to practise any of the exercises in this book, take a few moments to 'check in' with yourself. Always feel free to continue the practice if that feels best for you at the time.

✳️ If your body is not able to do any of the movement postures, just sit comfortably and run through them in your mind. Please never do anything that causes pain. Less is often more.

1
Being in the Now

Living moment by moment, and seeing
everything afresh without judgement
and worry lets us experience life rather
than simply get through it.

Look Around You and Live Longer

In this exercise, the invitation is to pick as a focus of awareness a new aspect of life. You may really look at a particular leaf on a tree, or a stone, flower or plant. You may want to think about a piece of furniture or decoration you like, wondering how it came into being and how many people were involved in its creation.

A recent study shows that mindfulness practices such as this may not only be responsible for structural changes in the brain, but also extend our life.

So far, the research has shown psychological and cognitive changes: improvements in perception and well-being, for example. However, it also appears that meditation might actually help delay the process of ageing by protecting the caps, or telomeres, located at the ends of our chromosomes.

With a sense of adventure and curiosity, we can learn and experience more, moment by moment

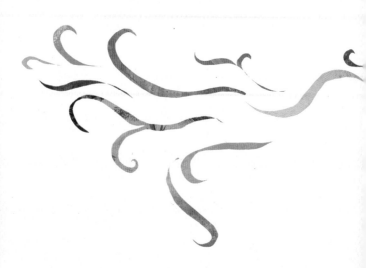

5 minutes

Awakening Your Breath

This important exercise helps us to breathe more fully, and strengthens and awakens us to face the day with confidence and calm. If you wish you can do it sitting on a chair or on the floor.

Stand in mountain pose
(see page 26), with the spine
lengthened upwards and the
legs and feet hip-width apart.
Position the arms by your
sides, palms to the front, so
the thumbs face outwards.

 Inhale and sweep/lift your
arms slowly up and overhead
until the hands meet above
the head, palms touching.
Exhale slowly as you lower
the arms back down to your
sides, moving slowly with your
breathing. See if you can deepen
and lengthen your breathing, and try
to feel the pause after each breath.

 Repeat 5–8 times.

Tune In!

The goal of any mindfulness practice is simply
to experience life as it unfolds. To stay present and
calm and not slip back into thinking/worrying mode,
we choose an anchor of awareness – a point of focus
we direct our mind to.

Here, you connect to sound, so that you can truly
experience the moment, and a whole lot of other moments,
with childlike curiosity and without judgement.

Start with 5 minutes and extend to longer sittings
if that feels right for you. Find a special spot in a quiet
part of your home or garden.

✳ Take a seat. Now gently close your eyes or keep
   them in soft focus (half-closed).

✳ Allow sounds to enter your awareness and to let them
   pass, like clouds passing by in the sky: sounds from
   near and far, coming and going. Let go of labelling
   sounds – a car, a bird, and so on – because as soon
   as we label, we tend to get involved in stories, which

trigger our left (thinking) brain, rather than our right (feeling) brain. All you need to do is be present to sound.

 You may notice that your hearing becomes more focused and that other brain activities seem to move into the background of your awareness. At other times, you may notice thoughts arising. This is the nature of the mind; it tends to get busy, even when we don't want it to. So, whenever you notice the mind wandering, gently and without judgement return your awareness, your mindfulness, to simply listening. This action is your anchor!

 You may notice after a few minutes that time seems not to matter any longer; your breathing may get longer and deeper, too. But even if 'nothing' happens and you think you are just sitting here, that is okay. Each practice will unfold differently and each person is unique. There is no right or wrong way of practising mindfulness.

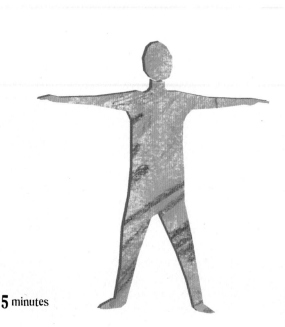

5 minutes

Standing Starfish

This pose gives you a feeling of being centred, with energy and confidence radiating from the navel region and spine into your arms and fingertips. It strengthens the legs, back, shoulders and arms.

Stand in mountain pose (see page 26), with arms at your sides, fingers pointing down.

 Step your feet apart with a toe-heel movement until they are about 50cm apart and parallel. Contract the pelvic floor in and up, and lengthen the spine upwards. Breathe and hold until you feel stable.

 Inhaling, lift your arms to a T-shape, palms facing down to the floor. Keep lengthening your spine upwards out of your pelvis and squeezing the sitting bones together ('pelvic floor lift') to pull the tailbone down. Relax the shoulders as you extend your arms and fingertips to the sides. Hold for 3–5 breaths.

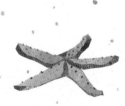

Feel the Earth: Mountain Pose

This simple yoga pose may help you be strong like
a mountain. Feeling connected to the earth lets
your body and mind exist in the here and now.
It also strengthens legs and improves posture.
As an alternative, imagine a mountain and feel
as strong and still as it does.

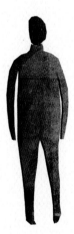

✳ Stand with feet hip-width apart, with arms by your side, palms facing in, gently touching the thighs.

✳ Take a few breaths to become aware of your breathing. When exhaling, contract the pelvic floor muscles and lift them up until you feel a squeeze at the base of your buttocks, a physical sensation as if your sitting bones are coming closer. This action supports the spine from below. Continue to breathe evenly. With the next exhalation, draw the entire abdominals to the spine and, at the same time, lengthen the spine upwards.

✳ Stand tall, with the spine straight and the head lifted. Breathe deeply and widely into the lungs, creating a sense of space in the entire chest area, with each in-breath. With the exhalation, roll the shoulders up, back and down, releasing any tension in the upper back.

✳ With each in-breath, feel the uplifting in the entire spine, and with each out-breath, as you gently draw the navel to the spine, feel the support you are giving your lower back.

Why Little Things Matter

Whatever you do as a daily practice can become your 'bell of mindfulness.' Step out of 'autopilot' and experience simple, routine tasks as if for the first time, savouring the sensations and absorbing the detail of the task you're focused on.

You may choose to:
~ Brush your teeth mindfully
~ Get dressed mindfully
~ Listen and talk mindfully
~ Eat and drink mindfully
~ Drive mindfully.

Many times I have heard people say: 'But I'll never get through all my chores if I slow down so much.' Maybe this is true. Maybe, however, by becoming more mindful, you may find new joy in everyday activities and eventually you may even be able to 'run' mindfully, that is, flow with focus through life.

2
Accept and Respond

Simple mindfulness practices engage
the mind and the body, helping you let go
and slowly bringing you back to a sense
of equanimity and peace.

Be with the Breath

Find a peaceful place. You can sit on a chair or on
the floor, or lean against a wall to support your spine.
Keep warm with a shawl or blanket around you.
You may wish to light a candle.

🌼 Focus on the sensations where your body contacts
the floor or chair. Exploring these sensations; simply
'feel' into your body and let it breathe itself.

🌼 Bring your attention to your chest and belly,
feeling them rise gently on the in-breath and fall
on the out-breath.

🌼 Be with each breath for its full duration. You may
even notice a short pause after each breath, and also
that each seems to have a life of its own.

**Minding the breath can be like
taming a wild horse. The aspiration is
to tame it with kindness and without
breaking its spirit**

Your mind may wander – thinking, daydreaming, planning or remembering – and lose touch with your breathing, but that is okay. Simply notice what it is that takes you away, then escort your focus back to your belly and the feeling of breathing.

 It is just as valuable to become aware that your mind has wandered and bring it back to the breath as it is to remain aware of the breath. After all, only a person being mindful will ever notice the wandering nature of the mind.

 At the end of your practice, please blow out the candle.

Tip ~ Try being with the breath at different times of the day: certain times may suit you better than others.

Roll Down for Serenity

In a process of 'letting go,' the roll-down stretches the muscles and helps release tension. It increases the mobility of the spine, stretches the back muscles, works the abdominals and stretches the hamstrings.

Feel peace at last!

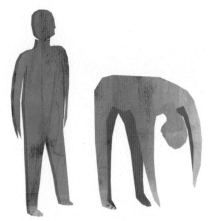

❈ Stand in mountain pose (see page 26), with your arms by your side.

❈ Lengthen your spine and, while breathing deeply, bring the chin to the chest and roll down as if rolling over a big ball. Your hands slowly glide down your thighs and help you control the movement. Go as far as you are comfortable; bend your knees. Draw in the abdominals a little.

❈ Hold for several deep breaths then slowly return. Exhale to squeeze the sitting bones together, draw the abdominals to the spine, then breathe in and out softly and deeply, straightening your spine as you roll up again, vertebra by vertebra, letting your head dangle, arms touching the legs to support the movement. Bring your head up last, rolling the shoulders back and down. Stand tall and be in control.

❗ *Avoid if you have a disc-related illness.*

'Talk' to Anger and Let It Go

Find a peaceful place and sit comfortably.
Wrap up in a blanket to keep warm and light
a candle if you prefer.

✳ Feel your feet firmly on the ground, rooted, your
buttocks and lower back supporting you, hands
resting in your lap. Let your facial muscles go loose.

✳ Notice your breath and allow your body to 'breathe
itself'. Sit and taste each breath when it enters your
body and observe how it leaves.

✳ When you are ready, experiment with mentally
moving towards your anger. It may be a barrage
of words or a feeling; it may have a colour or shape
or form. You may even feel, by allowing thoughts
about it to arise, that you are becoming a little more
agitated than before, but this is perfectly normal.

Now 'talk' to your anger, saying something like:
'I want to understand you. Let me experience you. Give me your all. I am just going to sit here and watch. I am not going to react and do what I would have done in the past.'

 Keep focusing on your breathing and 'dancing', as it were, with your anger.

 Continue this for a while and see how you experience 'being with' a discomfort. Remember, this too will pass. Finish the exercise when you feel the right moment has arrived.

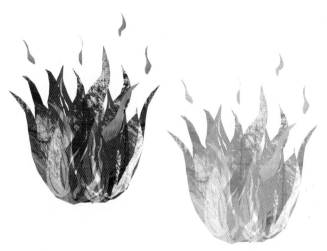

5 minutes

Do the Cat Stretch Six Times

We hold the tension of unresolved feelings in our bodies. The cat stretch can help to release mental and muscular tension in the back, spine, shoulders and neck, returning us to a state of calm awareness.

❋ If you are able, get on your hands and knees on a yoga mat, forming a box position with the wrists directly under your shoulders, and knees under the hips.

❋ Lengthen the spine from the top of the head to the tailbone. Inhale, and feel your belly moving away from the spine, then exhale, drawing your navel towards your spine. Repeat 3 times, drawing the belly/navel closer to the spine with each exhalation.

❋ Exhale, drawing your navel towards the spine, tucking the tailbone under and moving the chin to the chest, rounding the spine into a C-shape, as if you are dropping over a beach ball. Feel the position. Breathe in and out.

✳ Inhale and reverse the movement. Slowly release your belly towards the floor and elongate your spine into the neutral position. Still inhaling, lift the chest and breast bone forwards and up, and look up. Keep the arms strong and the shoulder blades back and down. Repeat the whole movement 6 times.

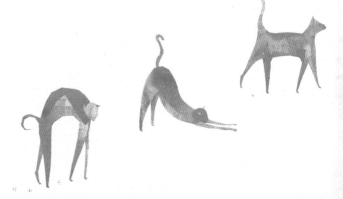

Tip ~ To protect your knees, place a cushion under them. If your wrists feel vulnerable, try rolling up the edge of the mat and placing them on it.

If you have a lower back problem and/or neck issues, start with a small movement and slowly increase the range of movement.

The Pebble Meditation

You can visualize a pebble or,
when in nature, you might choose
a real pebble and gently cast it
into the water as a mindful way to
connect with your inner sensations.

❋ Be comfortable on the floor or on
a chair, and imagine being at the
edge of a beautiful pond. The sun
is shining and you can see some of
its rays reflected in the water. There
are waterlilies, and blue and green
dragonflies circling. Maybe you hear
a frog croaking. Allow yourself to
visualize this pond in all its glory
and add any image or sound to
the picture that you create in
your imagination.

✳️ Now see yourself picking up a small, flat pebble and throwing it into the water, watching it sink a little. Notice what thoughts, feelings and sensations you are experiencing right now. Allow the pebble to sink deeper and see whether any sensations, images or feelings change.

✳️ Let the pebble settle at the bottom of the pond. You may even be able to see where it has settled. What do you feel, sense or think now? Are there any messages arising from your consciousness that you need to hear or bring to your awareness?

✳️ Stay a little longer and just breathe, from moment to moment… taking care of now.

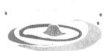

The Guest House

This being human is a guest house.
Every morning a new arrival.

A joy, a depression, a meanness,
some momentary awareness comes
as an unexpected visitor.

Welcome and entertain them all!
Even if they're a crowd of sorrows,
who violently sweep your house
empty of its furniture, still,
treat each guest honourably.
He may be clearing you out
for some new delight.

The dark thought, the shame, the
malice, meet them at the door
laughing, and invite them in.

Be grateful for whomever comes,
because each has been sent
as a guide from beyond.

Jalal Al-Din Rumi (1207–1273)
translated by Coleman Barks

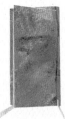

3
Making Your Mind Up

When we procrastinate and distract ourselves with 'busyness', we avoid engaging with the real thing — our lives. Mindfulness helps us become really present, so we respond wisely to a challenge and experience each moment as it unfolds.

Walking Mindfully

Experience the miracle of moving, of not needing
to get anywhere, with the ancient practice of walking
meditation. You can do this inside or outside, wherever
it is safe and protected, so you cannot trip over. A private
garden, no matter how small, is ideal. It's enough to be
able to walk 10 steps or so in one direction.

Practise mindful walking maybe for 10 minutes initially,
then expand it gradually to 20 minutes, should you
wish or need to.

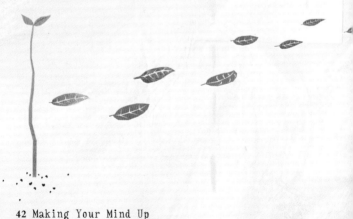

✳ First, take a stance to feel really connected to the
earth, feet hip-width apart and solidly rooted
to the ground. Take in the area you are to
walk in, keeping your eyes open and
looking straight ahead of you
and not down.

✳ Then, very slowly start to lift your right foot from
the ground. Notice the heel peeling off the ground,
and the weight shifting onto the left leg and foot.
Having peeled the right heel off, observe how you
are moving it forwards ever so slowly and gently
placing it down exactly one step ahead. While you
are placing the right foot down, you are observing
the left heel beginning to peel off the ground and
the weight shifting back onto the right leg.

❋ You may notice you are walking in a slightly wobbly way, as you have slowed down the pace so much. It may be helpful to imagine making real footprints in the ground, like walking on a sandy beach. Your awareness will be fully occupied with the lifting, shifting and placing of each foot step by step, as well as mindfully observing how your weight shifts from left to right and back again.

❋ When you have done approximately 10 steps in one direction, take your time in turning around. Notice how your hips swirl around very gradually and, before starting your next set of steps, stand once again mindfully rooted to the ground.

❋ With each passage you walk, it is possible to feel more and more grounded and safe, although each person's experience differs. Try to do it with an attitude of openness and curiosity, as would a child. Isn't it miraculous how the body knows exactly what to do?!

Try the 10-Step Walk

Here's a story about one of my clients who used mindful walking to de-stress at work. You might like to try out his method, too.

Tom likes to walk in the office. He can just about fit in 10 steps. At one end of the office there is a beautiful window looking out onto a luscious green bush; at the other end hangs a poster of his favourite city. So, should his mind wander off during the 10 steps, he is mindfully walking, these two images are reminders to bring him back to it. Each step he breaks down by mentally repeating 'lifting, shifting, placing.' He lifts the heel, shifts the foot forwards and then places it down. The focus on the soles of his feet and the repetitive instruction help him to centre and let go of all the fear-inducing aspects of his life.

5 minutes

How are You Feeling?
Check Your Breathing

By observing your breath,
you can make such a difference
to how you feel

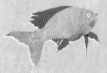

Breath is life energy. When we restrict our breathing, we diminish our life energy. Feeling agitated and indecisive is often accompanied by shallow breathing. Try this technique to enhance your breathing.

Deep breathing expands the lungs which then send a direct message to your heart, which in turn starts beating slower.

✳ Take a moment to get closer to your breathing – to 'befriend' it. Is it shallow or deep, slow or fast, smooth or rough, regular or irregular? Do you tend to push it or hold it? If you explore your breathing with this curiosity, you will get a good insight into where you are right now.

✳ From this baseline, you can notice any differences. If you continue to watch your breathing, you can experience a more energetic self and achieve joy and a zest for life again.

The Gentle Chest-Opener

This posture will help you very gently and compassionately to reverse the close-down posture (the foetal position) that often goes with low mood.

☀ Place a rolled-up bath towel on a blanket or yoga mat. Sit on the end of the blanket or mat and then, supporting yourself with your arms, lower your spine over the entire towel, from the tailbone to the top of the head.

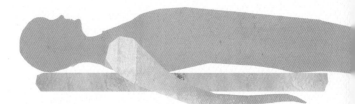

Your arms are by your sides, or extended in a T-shape. Your legs are bent or stretched; support the back of your legs with a rolled-up blanket if you need to. Relax the legs so they fall open. If your head needs support, use a pillow.

 You are now opening your chest, deepening your breathing. Stay here for 5–15 minutes.

 To finish, roll over onto your side and remove the towel to the side. Finally, roll over onto your back again and feel any sensations in your back and chest. It's likely that your chest will now feel a lot more spacious.

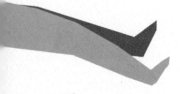

Do the Knee Hug

This is a wonderful way to release anxiety and
the feeling of containment offers a sense of focus.

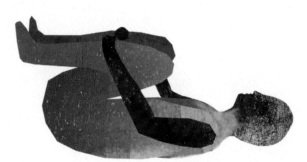

When you are in position, control and steady your breathing and create a sense of groundedness

 Begin in a relaxed, comfortable position,
lying on your back on a yoga mat or blanket.
If you need to support your neck, use a pillow
or rolled-up towel.

 Bend your legs, one after the other, into the chest
and gently hold them, but avoid pulling them, into
the chest. Keep your spine long as you press each
vertebra into the floor, and avoid hunching the
shoulders up. If you struggle to hug your legs,
hold them behind the knees. Pay attention to your
breathing. Hold for as long as you feel comfortable.

 When you are ready, gently let go of your knees and
relax your body into the floor.

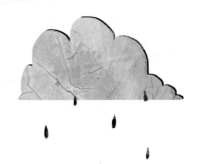

inspiration

An Invitation

When anxiety hovers above your light and shadows and all your actions, please do not fear them too much. I would like to remind you that life has not forgotten you. It is holding you by your hand and will not let you fall. Why do you want to shut out of your life any uneasiness or any depression? For after all, even though you do not know now where all of this will lead, these experiences may lead to the change that you were always hoping for.

From *Letters to a Young Poet*
by Rainer Maria Rilke
adapted by Patrizia Collard

4

Simply Be

Entering a state of 'being' rather than
'doing' can release us from the 'worry mind'
and help us taste each moment as it arises.
With this calmness, we can move towards
acceptance of how things are.

'Be' with the Body Scan

With this practice, we travel through our body to understand what it is trying to say to us and create a healthy relationship with a body that often we deem imperfect. This is the 'house' we live in, so it may be helpful to learn to accept it and make the most of it.

※ Make yourself comfortable. Lie on your back on a mat or rug, on the floor or on your bed. Cover yourself with a blanket and gently let your eyes close.

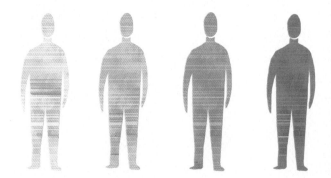

✳️ Take a few moments to get in touch with the movement of your breath and the sensations in your body. When you are ready, bring your awareness to the physical sensations in your body, especially touch, where your body is in contact with the floor or the bed. On each out-breath, allow yourself to let go, sinking a little deeper into the mat or bed.

✳️ Now bring your awareness to the physical sensations in the lower abdomen, to the changing sensations as you breathe in and out. It may be helpful to put your hand on your belly and to really feel each breath, noticing that some may be deeper, others shallower, and that there tends to be a little pause between each in- and out-breath.

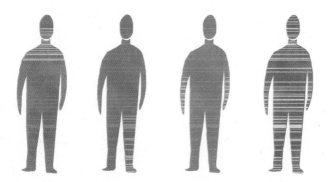

✳ Bring your focus gently down the left leg, into the left foot. Focus on each of the toes of the left foot – the big toe, the little toe and the toes in between, then the sole of the foot. Then continue to move your awareness further up your left leg, to the calf, the shin, the knee, the thigh.

✳ When you are ready, on an in-breath, feel the breath entering the nostrils, then the lungs, and then passing down into the abdomen, the left leg and the left foot. Then, on the out-breath, feel or imagine the breath coming all the way back up, out of the foot, into the leg, up through the abdomen and chest, and out through the nose. On each out-breath, have a sense of releasing any tension or discomfort. As best you can, continue this for a few breaths.

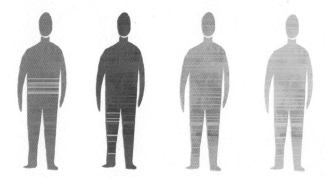

❈ Continue to bring awareness, and a gentle curiosity, to the physical sensations in each part of the rest of the body in turn. As you leave each major area, 'breathe into it' on the in-breath, and let go of that region on the out-breath.

❈ When you become aware of any tension or other intense sensation in a particular part of the body, 'breathe into it' and, as best as you can, have a sense of letting go, or of releasing, for the duration of the out-breath.

❈ After 'scanning' the whole body in this way, spend a few minutes being aware of a sense of the body as a whole, and of the breath flowing freely in and out of your body.

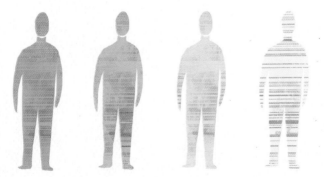

10 minutes

Do the Foot Scan

In this practice, we are trying to get the furthest away from our thinking mind, which is ruminating around 'attack' thoughts, and move into our 'feeling mind' to connect with our inner space. Keep your eyes shut or half-closed; you are not looking at your foot but simply attempting to bring awareness to it. It doesn't matter whether you are sitting or standing.

❋ Bring your awareness to your left foot. Really feel it with your mind, and slowly guide yourself through the territory of your foot with kind attention.

You could say:
'I am becoming aware of my left foot, my big toe, my little toe and all the toes in between, even the spaces between the toes, feeling them, sensing them…'

Or/and this:
'Now I am bringing awareness to the tips of my toes and to my toenails, then to the heel of my foot, the instep and the front part and now the whole sole of my foot.'

❋ Spending a good couple of minutes on your foot in this mindful way directs your conscious thinking away from the beliefs that had been feeding your anger or negative thoughts initially.
This may be enough that you can now further calm the mind with a walking or sound meditation, or with a mindful stroll
(see pages 42–44).

The Table Top: for when You are Ill

You can do this this simple co-ordination of breath
and movement from your bed to slowly bring back
some energy. When you get up, you can incorporate
simple tasks, such as going to the bathroom, getting
dressed, making a cup of tea, and so on, mindfully.

※ Lie on your back with your legs stretched out and
   allow yourself to be totally calm.

※ When inhaling, open your toes like a flower opening
   to the sunshine. When exhaling, scrunch your toes as
   if the flower is closing. (If you tend to get cramps,
   do the closing action very gently.)

※ Now when you are inhaling, softly point your toes
   away from you, and when exhaling, flex your feet.

※ Curl the ankles in each direction.

※ Bring one leg to table top position (the knee is
   bending at 90°). When you are inhaling, open the

knee and extend
the leg towards
the ceiling.
When exhaling,
fold it back to the
table top position. Change sides after 6–9 repetitions.

❋ Now bring your feet closer to the buttocks, one after
the other, and rest the feet on the bed, hip-width
apart. When inhaling, drop/open the knees to the
side, and when exhaling, bring the knees back up.

❋ With arms in a V-shape or a T-shape, exhale, dropping
both knees to the right; the hips, pelvis, lower back
and spine will follow, with the head staying soft in the
centre or turning slightly to the left. When inhaling,
hold the position. When you
begin to exhale, return the
spine, pelvis, hips and
knees back to the start
position. Repeat on
the other side.

❋ Do this gently, for as long as
you feel comfortable.

5 minutes

Being with Loss

How can we be in a wise relationship with pain, fear and loss? There is no simple answer. What I can share with you is an attempt to sit with 'what is.' Don't try to change it, to wish it away or 'fast forward'. This is perhaps the most fundamental mindfulness practice, and yet the most challenging for a 'quick-fix' society.

* Sit comfortably. Feel your feet firmly grounded on the floor, your back aligned with your neck and your hands resting in your lap.

* Focus on your breathing. Allow each in-breath to enter your body and expand for its full duration – don't force anything, just allow your body to breathe itself. Then, after a natural break, breathe out the out-breath for its full duration, until it comes to a natural end. Do this for a while, as long as it takes to feel settled enough.

* Then focus on the 'loss' – it may be health, a friendship or partnership, or the death of somebody close. Gently say: 'Whatever it is (here, you fill in the 'loss' verbally or as an image) let me feel it.' Start with a very simple phrase or image and just hold this in your awareness. Be with it, feeling, seeing the loss, facing it, even if it is painful, but don't pretend it is not there. You may only be able to do this for a minute or two. Let go of the thought or image, and return to the simple breath of life.

Accepting What Is

Taking a mindful approach to illness
means initially accepting what is.

Buddha told this story of the 'two arrows'
to his visitors:

*Life often shoots an arrow at you and wounds you.
However, by not accepting what has happened, by
worrying about it, by saying it is unfair and wondering
how long the pain will last, we tend to shoot a second
arrow into the open wound and increase and prolong
the pain. Pain is often a given, but suffering is optional.*

5
Mindful Eating

By truly noticing what we eat and drink,
we can cultivate gratitude for the food
we have. This gives us a sense of well-being
and peace, when we no longer need to use
food to fix our problems.

Eating with Pleasure

Frequently, we overeat because of stress hormones that float through our system. When we experience the fight-or-flight response, the body thinks it is in danger and needs fuel for all the extra tasks it may have to perform. To get that extra fuel, we crave sugar or carbohydrates, as they can easily be converted into energy.

Are you getting the picture? At times of great stress, it stands to reason that you will not have an urge to eat cucumbers or carrots, alas! The body cannot differentiate between real danger and perceived danger – even watching a horror film can set off the stress response. The body just does what it evolved to do 700,000 years ago.

Another trigger that lures us into eating more, but not necessarily wholesome, food is loneliness. Eating equals a sense of safety. Although reasons for disordered eating are beyond the realms of this book, I simply invite you to see if you can reintroduce pleasurable, mindful eating into your daily life. To really savour your food, you may want to experiment eating with a smaller fork from a smaller plate. Drinking liquid with a straw can help you feel calmer.

In the wild, a gazelle will never graze if a lion is on the prowl

5 minutes

Raisin Practice

This mindful eating practice will help you to reconnect to the pleasure in food. You can use a couple of raisins, or you might prefer small pieces of chocolate, some nuts or any quick snack food as an alternative. Make sure that you pause after each step.

~ Focus on this food and imagine you have never seen anything like it before.
~ Hold it in the palm of your hand.
~ Notice any differences in size, colour, form, weight and shape.

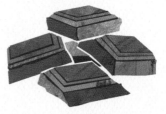

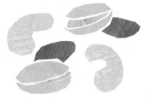

~ Look at the raisins even more carefully, observing the ridges and the surface.

~ Pick one up and explore its texture. Maybe squeeze it or pull it a little.

~ Examine the way the light is falling on it.

~ Let your sense of vision really have a feast.

~ If you start thinking 'Why am I doing this?' or 'This is silly', recognize those thoughts as random thoughts, and return your awareness, without judgement, to viewing.

~ Now smell the raisins, holding one just beneath your nose, and, with each in-breath, notice any aroma that may be there.

~ Place one of them near your ear, squeezing and rubbing it and checking whether a sound is apparent. Is there? Let yourself be surprised.

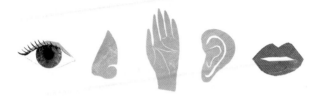

- ~ Now look again at the object and then gently touch the surface of your lips with one of them. Does that skin contact feel any different from the one you were experiencing when holding the raisin between the thumb and finger?
- ~ Slowly take the object towards your mouth, feeling your arm rising effortlessly to the right position, perhaps also feeling your mouth watering.
- ~ Gently place the food in your mouth without biting it. Notice how it is 'received', how the body knows exactly what to do, exploring the sensations of having it in your mouth.
- ~ When you are ready, very consciously take a bite into it and notice the flavours that are released.
- ~ Slowly chew it, noticing the saliva in your mouth and the change in consistency of the raisin. Observe anything that may be completely new to you.

Food should be savoured by the mind as well as the body

~ Then, when you feel ready, swallow the pulpy mass, seeing if you can first detect the intention to swallow as it comes up, so that even this is experienced consciously before you actually swallow it.

~ Finally, see if you can follow the sensations of swallowing, sensing the raisin moving down to your stomach, and also realizing that your body is now exactly one raisin fuller. What are you still tasting in your mouth? What is your tongue doing now? Is there a desire to eat a second raisin?

~ Engage with childlike curiosity and playfulness.

After this everyday practice, you may feel somewhat calmer and more settled. Just imagine if you ate each spoonful of a meal – not every meal but maybe one a day – in the same manner. Alternatively, you could try eating an apple or drinking your favourite drink in this way.

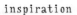 inspiration

Make Tea a Ritual

The twentieth-century Viennese writer Peter
Altenberg tells the following story about the
joy and deep satisfaction of drinking tea:

*Six o'clock in the evening is approaching. I can sense it drawing near.
Not quite as intensely as children feel Christmas Eve, but creeping
up all the same. At six o'clock on the dot I drink tea, a celebratory
enjoyment devoid of disappointment in this ailing existence. Something
that makes you realize that you have the power of calming happiness
in your hands. Even the action of pouring fresh water into my beautiful,
wide half-litre nickel kettle gives me pleasure. I wait patiently for it to
boil, listening out for the whistling sound, the singing of the water.*

*I have a huge, deep, round mug made of red-brick-coloured Wedgwood.
The tea from Café Central smells like meadows in the countryside.*

The tea has a golden yellow hue, like fresh hay. It never gets too brown, but remains light and delicate. I drink it mindfully and very slowly. The tea has a stimulating effect on my nervous system. Everything in life seems to be more bearable and lighter thereafter.

Drinking my tea at six o'clock never seems to lose its power over me. Every day I long for it as intensively as the day before, and when I drink it I lovingly embrace it into my being.

Translated and adapted by Patrizia Collard
from *Sonnenuntergang im Prater*
by Peter Altenberg

Nourishing the Body: Revisiting the Body Scan

On pages 54–57, we practised the body scan journey lying down with the legs falling open. This time we choose a posture that is more alert, and we focus mainly on the torso to really get in touch with those areas of the body that help us feel connected to the process of nourishment.

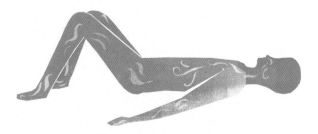

Tip ~ Prop your head up with a pillow and try not to fall asleep. The intention of the body scan is to stay awake to the experience of being alive.

❋ Begin by sitting on a chair, or lie down with knees bent in a triangle position.

❋ Start with your head and bring awareness to the crown, the back and the forehead.

❋ Bring awareness to your entire face, then your neck and shoulders, arms and hands, buttocks, legs and feet. Feel that your feet are firmly grounded on the floor.

❋ Now bring alertness to your torso: the back, the spine, the chest and then the abdomen. Notice how the breath moves in and out of your body, with particular focus on those areas that rise and fall with the breath.

❋ Now to your digestive organs: the stomach and the colon. Rest with awareness here. Gently remember that this is where all nourishment is received and digested. The energy created through this process is now fuelling your whole body. Smile into these areas, bringing awareness and gratitude to them and, on each in-breath, allow oxygen to flow into them, and release any tension, discomfort or critical thoughts on the out-breath.

❋ Stay for a while with the breath in this part of your body until you feel a sense of calm and kindly appreciation.

Mindful Eating Every Day

Each meal of the day can be a call to mindfulness and gratitude. If possible, and without a sense of duty, recall how many steps were necessary to create, for example, the lovely soup in the bowl in front of you.

Freely connect to the gardeners who planted and harvested the vegetables, the potter who created the bowl, the cook who prepared the meal. Really taste the dish and see whether you can guess how many ingredients went into it. The simplest meal can become a feast with a little 'dash' of awareness.

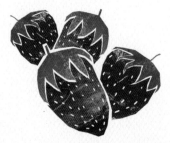

6
Gratitude and Compassion

Gratitude and mindful self-compassion
can heal and bring peace to you. Gratitude
comes when we are mindful, observing the
simple beauty in our lives.

Gratitude Practice: Write It Down

Gratitude and appreciation help us turn towards joy and gladness, which create chemicals of well-being and peace in our whole body.

Studies show that the regular practice of gratitude and appreciation, including writing down the experiences you feel grateful for, can lead to better health, less stress and a more optimistic outlook on life.

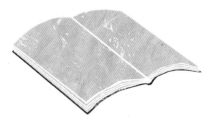

❋ Find a peaceful spot where you can sit
 down and write in a notebook and meditate.

❋ Give yourself a few minutes and note down all
 the things you are grateful for (such as friendships,
 things about yourself, your body, home, pleasurable
 memories, and so on.)

❋ Read through your list and internally give words of
 thanks to each point you noted. For example: 'Thanks
 for my beautiful smile, thanks for my special favourite
 mug, my last holiday…' When you give thanks, really
 tune into all five senses as best as you can.

❋ Bring awareness to this moment. What are you
 grateful for right here and now? How does this
 feel in your body, and where do you feel it? Gently
 breathe and sit with gratitude for a little while longer.

The Big 'I' – Self-Compassion

Self-compassion can be the yin to the yang of
mindfulness. We need to be kind and accepting
of ourselves when we don't manage to be mindful,
while we need mindfulness to observe our own
self-critical behaviour and thoughts.

❊ Take a large sheet of paper and draw on it a big letter
'I'. The big 'I' represents you as a whole, all the
actions you've ever done, all aspects of your body,
mind and talents, and so on.

❊ Over one week, write down, within the big 'I', little
'i's, whenever they arise – choose one coloured pen
for what you like about yourself, and another colour
for what you feel needs improving or accepting.
Make each little 'i' represent one aspect only. So,
I would write in green: 'enjoys meeting people',
'good at cooking', 'nice eyes'. Then I would put
in red: 'increase patience' and 'improve organization'.

❋ It is wonderful to really see, in large scale, how we consist of a broad choice of behaviours and characteristics. Nobody will be either a complete failure, or perfect.

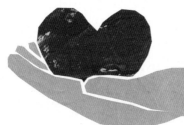

This is our human condition,
and to accept it fully
is the starting point
for change

Metta Meditation: Loving Kindness

Metta is usually translated as 'loving kindness'. By
practising it, you may find you are able to deal with
situations with greater ease and lightness. I truly feel
that it is a very empowering tool for transformation.

You can visualize, in the centre of your chest, your
'emotional' heart, an image of yourself as you are now or
how you were as a child, perhaps supported by a loving
other. If visualizing is difficult, try just seeing your name
written in the centre of your heart.

The metta practice starts with the pure intention
that we wish to increase self-compassion from within.
We may use the analogy of planting a seed, which
we 'tend' through the practice until it grows into
a beautiful flower or tree.

'May I be safe and protected.'
'May I be peaceful.'
'May I live at ease and with kindness.'

In week two, after meditating on ourselves, we add
somebody we love and care for:
'May you be safe and protected.'
'May you be peaceful.'
'May you live at ease and with kindness.'

Week by week we can expand the practice.

We finally go still further, to include people we
hardly know, or people who may have caused us
irritation or hurt:
'May all beings be safe and protected.'
'May all beings be peaceful.'
'May all beings live at ease and with kindness.'

With this practice, we start with the mere intention
of loving kindness, but experience has shown me that
persisting with it can wonderfully enrich our lives.
If every one of us just managed to touch one 'other'
through this practice, the world would indeed be
a safer, kinder and a more peaceful place in which
to live.

Smile into the Body: a Brief Sitting Practice

This 'smile' softens the body and brings an almost instant sense of calm. Begin by adopting a comfortable, dignified sitting posture in a quiet space.

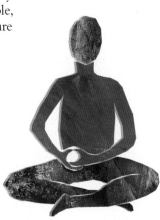

Allow any thoughts —whether bad or good — to pass you by like a cloud in the sky

※ Join the hands with both thumbs, and the fingers of one hand resting in those of the other.

※ Focus on your breathing. Let each breath unfold by itself, neither lengthening it, nor expanding and deepening it. Allow the body to breathe itself, and pay witness to this miraculous breath, coming and going.

※ When you feel settled, having breathed like this for a few minutes, allow a gentle smile to arise on your face. Notice how it softens all the facial muscles and how, breath by breath, this softening and relaxing moves further and further into every cell of your body. Soon your whole body will be a gentle, soft smile.

※ Sit with this for a while and simply 'be', moment by moment.

When we have genuine self-love we can tap into our true goodness, see the gifts we've been given and then experience the joy of sharing them with others

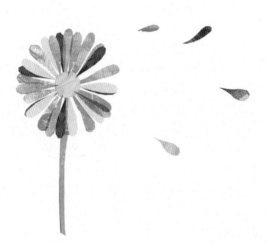

7
Everyday Mindfulness

Mindfulness is an attitude rather
than a skill. Whenever we feel we have
reconnected to the old treadmill of 'autopilot',
we may choose, if we wish, to step out
and start again, making our everyday
lives more pleasurable, and present.

A Mindful Day

※ On waking, you may focus for a little while on your breathing, just observing it with gentle curiosity. You may want to smile into your body before getting up, breathing gently into every part. Continue having a mindful bath or shower, brushing your teeth with awareness and mindfully getting ready for the day.

※ Some people like to meditate in the morning, others in the evening or even at different times of the day. However, it is a good idea to pencil this special 'meeting with yourself' into your diary.

※ You may decide to do breathing practices a few times a day, maybe every time you wash your hands or enjoy a drink; and when you eat and drink, do so with mindful gratitude.

※ Communicating with others is another wholesome part of the practice. Listen to yourself answering the phone or having a conversation. Are you mindful of how you speak and listen, giving space to the other person and choosing words with honesty but without the need to win or score points?

✳ When there are moments that might in the past have amounted to nothing or to frustration, such as being stuck in traffic, you could try to breathe mindfully, or listen to music – really listen – or simply take in your surroundings, really seeing life as it presents itself at that given moment.

✳ When the day is coming to an end, you may want to note down in a diary your 'EGS' of the day: what did you Enjoy today, what are you Grateful for and what are you Satisfied with? This could be something as mundane as having made a particular phone call or paid a bill; just a little action is enough. Before switching off the light, you are once again invited to connect to your body with kindly awareness, smiling and breathing into it.

Listen to yourself answering the phone or having a conversation

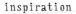

A Daily Meditation

Let us be still for a few moments,
without moving even our little finger
so that a hush descends upon us.
There would be no place to go,
nor to come from, for we would
have arrived in this extraordinary moment;
there would be a stillness and silence,
that would fill all of our senses,
where all things would find their rest.
Everything would then be together in a deep connection,
putting an end to 'us and them', this against that;
we would not move in these brief moments,
for that would disturb this palpable presence;
there would be nothing to be said nor done,
for life would embrace us in this wondrous meeting,
and take us into its arms as a loving friend.

Christopher Titmus

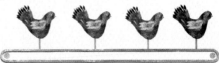

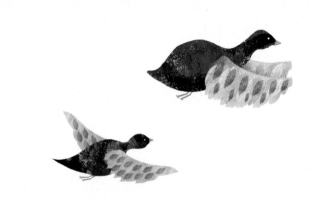

Moments

Less than a second
The universe was born
The stars we see so clearly
Seem only a little far
Almost untouchable
But not quite
A seed breaks open
A new life
Moments
Here now
But briefly

Patrizia Collard

Turning a minus into a plus

A client who attended one of my courses
told me right at the end that 'everyday
mindfulness' had changed her life. What
had really turned her life around was
changing her attitude to something
she had to do every day, and had
despised until recently.

She had read research papers that indicated that
mindfulness had very beneficial effects on skin
disorders. She suffered from severe eczema, controlled
only by a rigid regime of applying cream to her
entire body, morning and night.

Although initially a little disappointed not to
be miraculously healed of her disease, she then
accepted that this was still an option, which might
happen one day soon or slowly over time.

She realised that one thing she could do now was
to apply the cream mindfully to each part of her
body, not rushing it, breathing gently into every
part she was attending to, and also bringing
a sense of gratitude for the fact that
this regime actually kept
the disease under control.
It became a kindly ritual
with a very different energy,
rather than the hugely disliked
ordeal it had been before.

What could you
do differently?

Peace

There is only silence
On the mountain tops
Among the tips of the trees
You perceive barely a breath
Even the birds in the forest
Keep still and are silent
Wait then
Just a little while longer
And you too
will find peace at last.

J.W. von Goethe
translated by Patrizia Collard

A Final Message

This little book is coming to an end, yet it is really only the beginning of another chapter, another adventure. I hope this book has helped you be inspired to live your life moment by moment, knowing that the only thing we can be certain of is that everything changes all the time.

Day by day I am more certain that any one of us is like a beautiful diamond that only needs a little bit of cutting here and there before it sparkles all over. An uncut diamond tends to look just like any stone, yet beneath that surface lies miraculous clarity and beauty.

With blessings,
Patrizia Collard

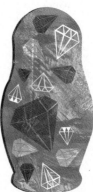

Acknowledgements

To Helen Stephenson, who suggested and
contributed to the physical exercises in this
volume. I feel honoured that she shared so
much with me. Thank you to Christopher Titmus
for allowing me to use his Daily Meditation,
and to the wonderful Coleman Barks, for
his translation of Rumi's *The Guest House*.

To Dan, Toby, Bernhard and Tybalt.

Thank you to all at Octopus – particularly
Abi Read for her beautiful illustrations and
Liz Dean, Consultant Publisher at Gaia Books,
who has been there every step of the way.

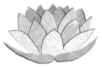